Longevity Through Naturopathy

Tips and Techniques to Keep Young Longer

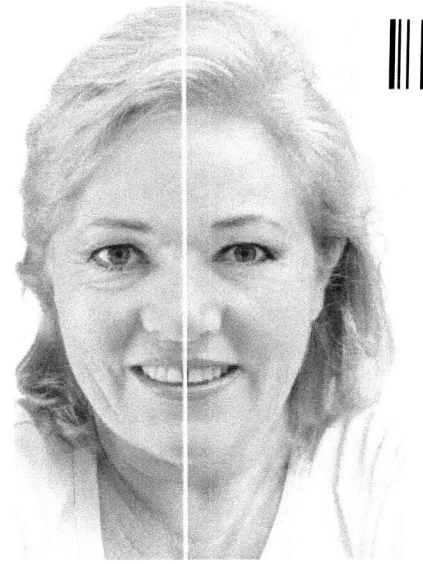

Health Learning Series

Dueep Jyot Singh

Mendon Cottage Books

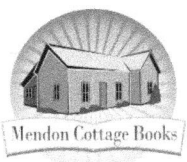

JD-Biz Publishing

Disclaimer

The information is this book is provided for informational purposes only. It is not intended to be used and medical advice or a substitute for proper medical treatment by a qualified health care provider. The information is believed to be accurate as presented based on research by the author.

The contents have not been evaluated by the U.S. Food and Drug Administration or any other Government or Health Organization and the contents in this book are not to be used to treat cure or prevent disease.

The author or publisher is not responsible for the use or safety of any diet, procedure or treatment mentioned in this book. The author or publisher is not responsible for errors or omissions that may exist.

Warning

The Book is for informational purposes only and before taking on any diet, treatment or medical procedure, it is recommended to consult with your primary health care provider.

Our books are available at

1. Amazon.com
2. Barnes and Noble
3. Itunes
4. Kobo
5. Smashwords
6. Google Play Books

Table of Contents

Introduction to Aging

They tell us that Methuselah lived 900 years. But then at that time longevity was the rule and not the exception. This process of growing old chronologically is a normal process of life. It occurs in every living thing present in nature. External factors also age nonliving things with the passage of time. A person is called old on the basis of his chronological age. That is why in the 21st century, anyone who has passed the age of three score and 10 will be considered to be old. However, in olden times, people lived for anywhere between 200 to 300 years, and still managed to look youthful and had as much energy as young adults.

The slowing down of the aging process is due to many factors, most of which are not present in the 21st century scenario. This includes clean-air, healthy pollution free atmosphere, a good natural diet, lots of exercise, and also a strong disease-free gene line.

With the passing of time, the natural good health and comparatively long age enjoyed by man 5000 years ago, has deteriorated a lot. The functional state of a living organism which is also known as the biological age is going to have a great influence on the aging of the person. This is going to show up mentally and physically in signs. Bring off the hair on the scalp is one such feature. Another feature is the presence of wrinkles and folds on the face, forehead, neck and forearms.

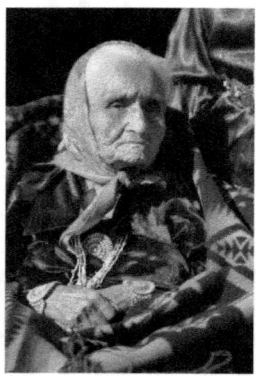

Aging is a natural process, but it can be restricted through naturopathy and natural tips and techniques.

The mental aging process is going to show up in different ways like age-related problems like memory loss, loss of concentration, weakness in the muscular frame, and tissue and digestive problems.

Individuals grow old at different rates. There are some races where people do not consider themselves to be old until they are in their 70s and 80s. On the other hand, there are other races, and individuals who begin to show the signs of aging while still in their 30s and 40s. The factors which cause the declining of these organ systems are many. Stress, strain, bad diet, lack of exercise, living in an polluted atmosphere are some of the modern day factors which do not contribute to longevity.

The effects of age are manifold. Your bladder capacity is going to be reduced. Urinary incontinence normally starts to trouble people as they grow older. Your kidneys are going to become less effective, and their toxin extracting capacities is going to decline. With the passing of time, you may find yourself forgetting things because the brain has started to lose cells. Some brain cells may get damaged.

From 40 onwards, people start feeling their age by a stiffness in their joints. That is because the cartilage of these joints are not as supple as they were when you were in your 20s. This stiffness is also going to be apparent in your neck area due to your spinal cord bones getting arthritic and stiff.

Exercise can prevent this from happening to a large extent. A sedentary lifestyle without any sort of exercise means that your muscle mass is going to decline with the passage of time.

Aging has a powerful psychological effect on the physical, mental, and spiritual well-being of human beings. However, it has been found out that the aging process in the last 500 years is premature aging due to environmental conditions, change of diet, and other factors affecting the body, spirit and mind.

Your body systems are programmed by nature to last 6 to 7 times as long as it normally takes an average person to reach the age of maturity. The people of olden days knew this natural truth. That is because their lifestyle followed a balanced and healthy diet, regular elimination of toxins and other waste products from the body, adequate rest of mind and body, keeping himself busy, both physically and mentally, avoidance of stress and tension, and continued expansion of experience, wisdom and knowledge. Along with that, spiritual and mental strength as well as a healthy and optimistic mental outlook was also called in to support physical longevity.

Introduction to Naturopathy

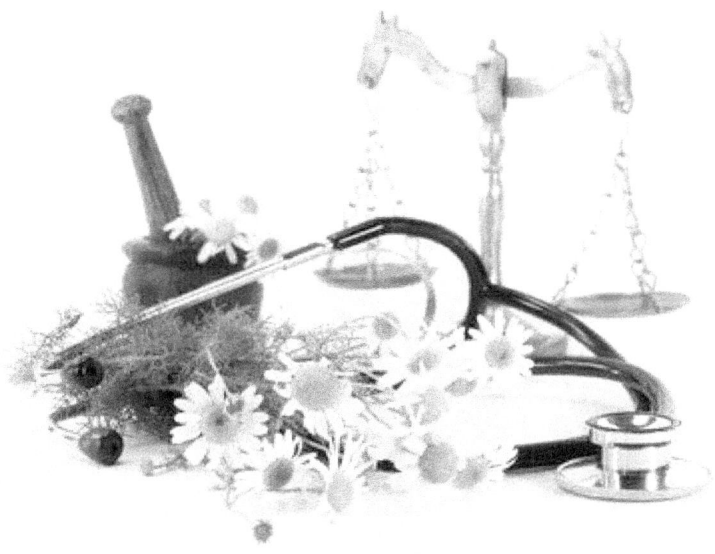

Naturopathy is an alternative system of traditional medicine, which is based on curing diseases and ailments the natural way. Exercise, proper diet, herbs, fresh fruit and vegetables, massage, aromatherapy and other traditional healing methods are used in naturopathy. Drugs are not use here at all, especially 21st-century chemical-based drugs.

Naturopathy has been long used as the traditional way to cure illnesses in the East and in the West for millenniums. The science of naturopathy concentrates on a few factors which are going to influence your future state of aging, lifestyle and general health as you grow older.

Humans generally want to believe that the aging process will automatically result in loss of organic functions, poor health, a slower metabolism, and mental faculties, and the development of old age-based diseases like cataract, diabetes, heart problems and arthritis.

This is so not true. Modern research has proven that longevity can be achieved through natural methods, including good nutritional diet and practice. This of course is the rehashing of information and knowledge. Our ancestors knew millenniums ago that slowed down the process of aging, but the 21st-century mind needs to have it in writing. After a lot of research has been done and a number of doctors with plenty of alphabets behind their names declared that yes, good diet and plenty of exercise and other naturopathic factors can have a rejuvenating effect on you, that is when you start to believe that yes, what the doctor said is true.

So take it from me. I'm not a doctor. I don't need to spend millions of tax owners hard-earned money on futile research to prove facts which already are known to make it more palatable to a credulous audience.

Instead, try some of my tips, based on the wisdom of the ages and experience.

Longevity Tips

You need to do a complete change in your lifestyle, and practice some physical, and mental rules in order to control the aging process. Some people say that you are only as old as you feel, how come a person who is 60 years old, doesn't look as old as she should be?

Look at that particular 60-year-old's outlook towards life. She has a positive outlook and has learned to accept old age gracefully. She doesn't create stress and tension in her family, looking for the latest miracle cure-all beauty treatment, which is going to make her look 30 years younger. That unfortunately is one of the multimillion dollar marketing strategy marketed by beauty companies selling their expensive products to people who cannot accept the fact that they are going old and gray.

Healthy habits when cultivated since young can slow down the aging process. This includes eating natural foods and undertaking exercises throughout your lifetime. This exercise routine is going to consist of walking about in the fresh air, getting your metabolism to work, eating more organic fruits and vegetables, and walking a lot.

I remember a time when I used to live in the mountains and walking 18 km a day did not seem to be much of a burden, because one was so used to doing that. And believe me, I never felt the need to go to a doctor up to my 30s until I had to move to a city and these walking habits dwindled away into nothingness.

It took three years for my health to deteriorate and start going downhill. That was because I was breathing in traffic fumes and eating food which had been preserved and packaged instead of eating natural stuff. My job may have been very well paying, but the stress and tension pertaining to responsibility of the senior management level added to the aging process. So the day I saw my first white hair at the age of 40, I decided enough was enough, and came back to the mountains.

Back to nature, back to natural foods, back to plenty of fresh air and exercise, plenty of laughter, a stress-free life and lots of rest, – along with short afternoon naps – and plenty of creative hobbies, pursuits, and activities which kept me busy and happy and there I was, my once rapidly aging process had slowed down. My contemporaries are all suffering from ulcers and wrinkles and potential heart problems. Even though they are rich and successful, they cannot get out of the rat race. They do not know how to relax. Their exercises limited to three days in the gym is not quite enough to keep them healthy and fit.

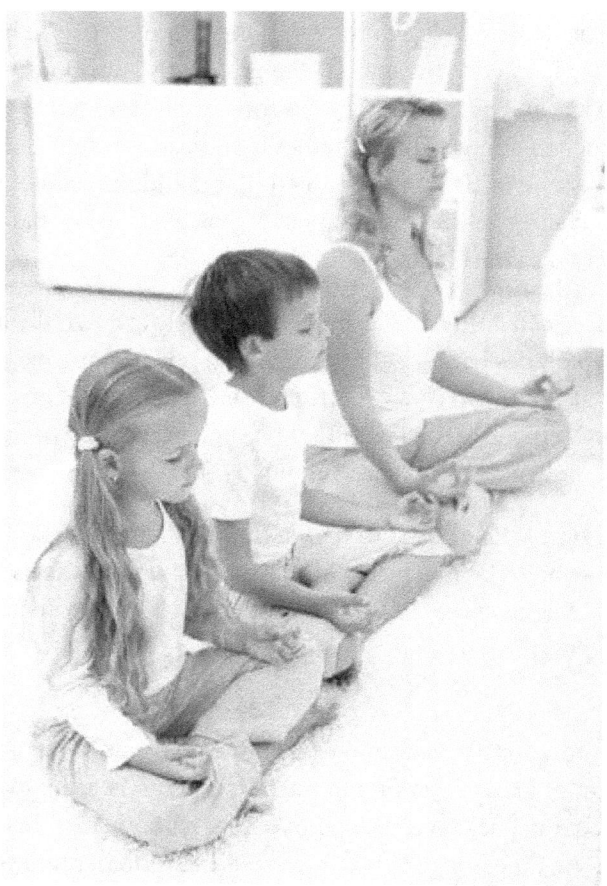

Meditation is one way in which you can gain mental tranquility and peace. These youngsters are starting young!

Somebody asked me the ancients secret in the East, with which they kept healthy, and I told them that in ancient India and in other Eastern countries, The lifespan of man was divided into four parts – childhood, and youth, where he gained knowledge and trained for a profession, adult age when he settled down and raised a family and the last stage – Vanaprastha when a person gives up all my digital desires and wants, and retreats to lead a life which is more spiritually inclined. A human being in this stage of life leaves the material world behind for his descendants and spends the rest of his life, concentrating on his own spiritual growth without any tension.

Such a person is not going to brood over past events, not worry about future events. He is just going to concentrate on the present moment and what is happening to him and around him at that particular moment. Such people were realistic in their expectations of their relationships with their adult and grown-up children. They had accepted the way they conducted their lives and their life choices.

The older generation at this time was used as a source of knowledge and experience. People came to them for advice, because that advice was given sparingly, and that advice was implemented because it was for one's own good.

However, nowadays this stage of spiritual withdrawal from the material world is practiced only in some parts of the East, where people of one generation lived together, being taken care by younger people who considered it an honor to do so in exchange for knowledge and wisdom of the ages. But as time went by this tradition started disappearing from the social fabric of mankind. One could consider this to be due to social upheaval and political unrest. Sanctuaries for old people were not considered feasible by people already on the move who needed to disappear during the night when information of invaders percolated through the word-of-mouth grapevine. And so the eldest generation was taken along with the family and still had to continue living in a material world with the family.

That is the reason why these sort of sanctuaries disappeared in the Middle Ages in many parts of the world. Nevertheless, up to 60 years ago, there was a tradition in the northeast part of the Indian subcontinent, where an old and sickly member of the tribe was taken to a fruit orchard and placed in a shelter. There he could eat fruit to his hearts content and breathe in the fresh air. Then the sun and the air were given the responsibility to rejuvenate and revitalize this ailing person.

He was visited twice a day by the youngest member of his family, who looked to his physical needs, and brought hot, nutritious homemade food for him. He was also brought large contents of fresh meat soup, fresh milk and milk products like butter and cheese, green vegetables and herbs. He was kept away from the daily tensions of his family, thus reducing the amount of stress and strain on his psyche. And 99% of the time, the person came back to his family, healthy, and sound. Naturopathy had worked her magic on him.

These hermitages in orchards are still being used to help people suffering from ailments as well as people who are feeling the aftereffects of old age.

Let me tell you about one of these herbs which were extensively grown in India and China to bestow longevity on their users. One was Ginseng.

Ginseng

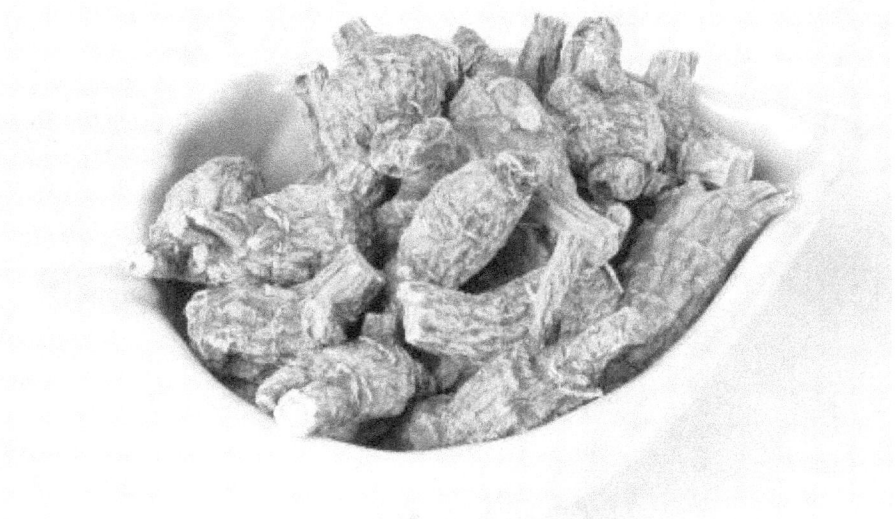

This wonder herb has been used extensively in Japan, Korea, China, Southeast Asia and India for its revitalizing and restorative power and as a remedy for a number of ailments for over 5000 years!

This was because it was well-known that ginseng taken regularly would have an extraordinary effect upon the taker's metabolism. It would also dramatically improve the general tone and quality of their system.

Ginseng is used in various ways. The dry and hard root is often sliced into pieces and steamed for about 5 to 10 minutes. It is then chewed. It can also be grated and powdered and then taken in doses of half a teaspoon mixed in a cup of boiling water with a little bit of cinnamon added for flavoring. You can also mix ginseng powder in fresh fruit juice, stir it well and drink it down for breakfast.

Alfalfa

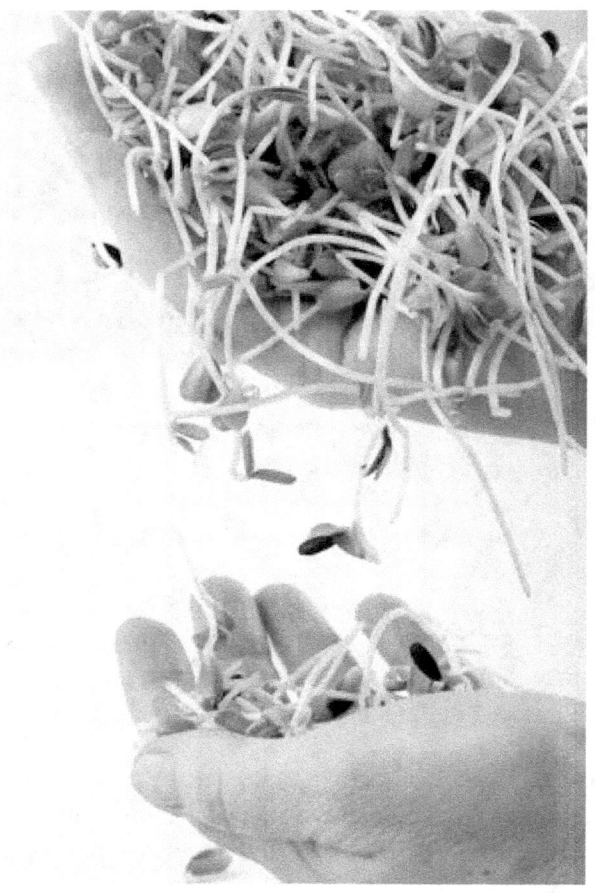

One doesn't know when people began to find that the nutritional and versatile Alfalfa promoted longevity. The stems, leaves, and the seeds were used to provide valuable nutrients to human beings, as well as animals. The Arabians called it the father of all foods. This grass is an extremely valuable source of vitamins A, B, D, E and G. It also has vitamin K, calcium, magnesium, sodium, potassium, chlorine, phosphorus and silicon.

The most beneficial property of alfalfa is that it has natural chlorophyll in abundance being a grass. Alfalfa in juice form has been used traditionally to cure heart diseases, trouble with the arteries, and in respiratory disorders. If you are pestered by plenty of stomach disorders, start eating alfalfa seed sprouts. A seed infusion is used for the treatment of high blood pressure and arthritis.

Bee pollen

Now this is a really surprising food which has been overlooked by people interested in naturopathy. We know all about honey, but we have overlooked the fine pollen grains yellow in color, in the supposedly waste product found inside the bottom of a beehive. This is processed bee pollen, which was originally collected from the blossoms of herbs and flowers.

According to the ancient texts of China, Persia, Egypt and Babylon, this remarkable substance of which is the secrets were only known to beekeepers has the magic key to the secret of continuous health, strength and longevity.

Even now many primitive types who still look on herbs and natural remedies know all about the power of the pollen grain. These grains consist of fats, protein, minerals, vitamin B complex, vitamins A, D, E, D, and free amino acids.

In 1945 a Russian researcher found a village in deep Russia where the people lived long and healthy lives, even though they had crossed the hundred year age limit. So he began to find out the secret of their longevity. He soon found out that the powerful matter produced by the bees, when they had made honey and which had dropped on the bottom of the beehive was a mixture of pure pollen and honey. This was eaten by them regularly and every day since childhood.

And they had learned the secret of longevity and good health.

Brahmi- Bacopa

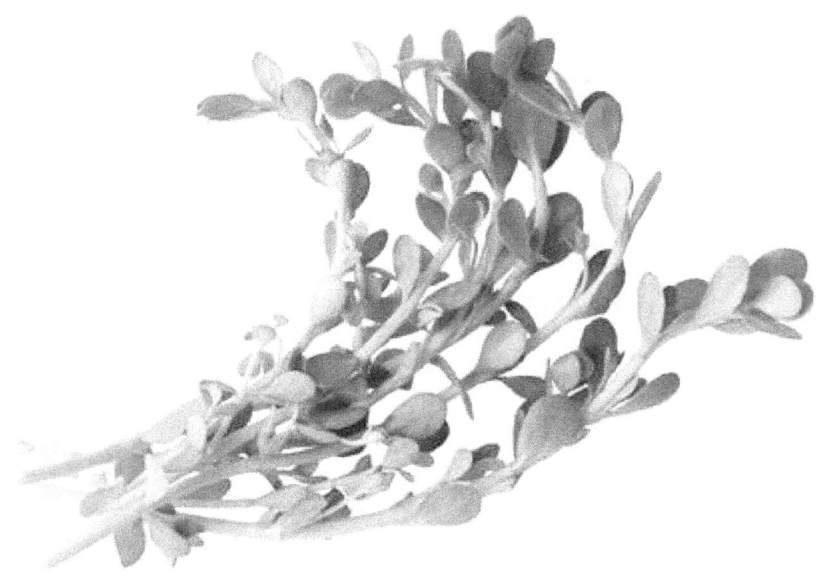

I'm now going to tell you about an Indian herb called Brahmi. [Bacopa monneira or Bacopa scrophulariaceae, or Bhrahmi booti (herb.)] It is also known as water hyssop in the West.

This herb is generally found in moist and wet places, such as the borders of water channels, bells and irrigated fields. The herb is used traditionally as a cardiac and nervous tonic and to purify the blood. It is a very powerful medicine, and that is why you just take the amount of root powder which sticks to the head of a pin with milk to cure yourself.

This herb has been known to cure it nervous disorders, rheumatism, loss of memory, and urinary problems which are conditions associated with old age.

But ancient medicine uses it as the best herb for longevity. Its regular use increases vitality, strengthens the various organs of the body and help to fight old age and diseases.

More than 500 years ago, a Chinese physician named Jinchigiyan started eating a mixture of ginseng along with *just two leaves of this plant* every day. He lived up to 250 years and would have lived even longer if he hadn't been killed in an invasion.

In many parts of the East, this herb is considered to be the cure-all for all kinds of diseases and to bestow longevity on its user. I normally use it to improve my memory. This is also very good amnesia cure.

 Drink this in your 40s and 50s and never bother about Alzheimers ever again, when you grow older.

- 20 g Bhrahmi booti powder

- Six tablespoons almond oil

- 3 g pepper

- 3 g crushed cardamom seeds

Mix these ingredients together. Now this happens to be a very powerful medicine. So you have to drink, just the amount which you put upon two pinheads (.22 grams!) with milk every morning and see your memory improving by leaps and bounds.

Fresh sheep liver is also excellent for curing **memory loss**.

Also, here is another use for this herb – it cures migraine completely, without you bothering about migril or vasograin tablets.

Drink a mixture of 5 grams bhrahmi booti and two grams of rock candy fried in ghee [clarified butter] and then swallowed with milk to cure your **migraine** permanently. You can drink this as long as you like, but you can be sure that this painful headache is going to be cured. At the same time, you'll be drinking milk regularly, isn't it?

Brahmi booti also cures **epilepsy**, completely.

- 10 g of Bhrami juice taken with 10 g of honey for 15 days will cure epilepsy completely. Don't take my word for it. This is a well-known ancient traditional timeworn remedy given to epileptic patients in the East.

Diet foods/supplements for longevity

Many of us do not eat almonds or dry fruit every day, possibly because they are so expensive, or possibly because we're not used to eating nuts, seeds, and other such foods, which prevent mental, and physical senility and prolong youthful vitality and appearance.

Here are some foods which you need to add to your daily diet to prevent you from aging. I begin with almonds, because not only are they an extremely good and nutritious dried fruit supplement to your diet, but almond oil is also capable of keeping your skin looking youthful and healthy for a long time.

Almonds

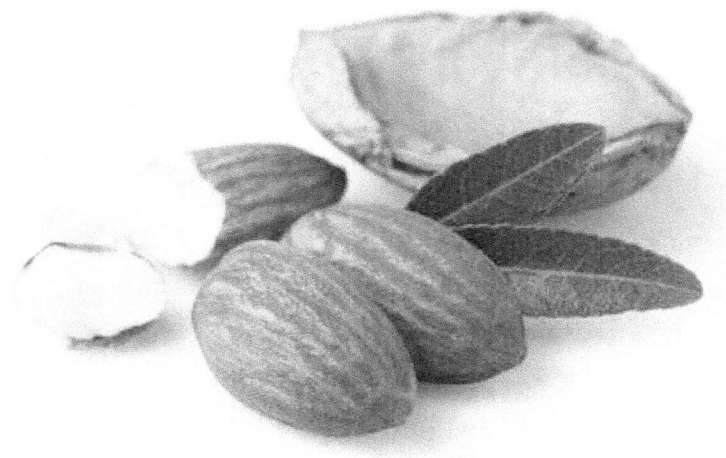

Almonds have been long called the king of nuts since ancient times, because it is rich in all the essential elements needed to keep your body healthy and strong. This is a valuable food remedy for curing you of several common problems, including anemia, constipation, skin disorders and respiratory diseases. It has been used to keep one's skin youthful looking for millenniums by peeling off the top brown skin and grinding the nuts into a paste with water. Then apply it all over your face. Not only is this going to have a bleaching effect on your face, but it is also going to keep your skin younger looking, thanks to the oil present in it.

Almonds have a number of chemical substances like copper, iron, phosphorus and vitamin B-1, which are necessary in the formation of new blood cells and hemoglobin. They also play a major role in maintaining the healthy and smooth physiological functions of your nerves, brain, hearts, bones and liver.

Longevity can be obtained with a regular diet of five almonds per day. It is going to preserve the vitality of your brain and strengthen your muscles.

Apples

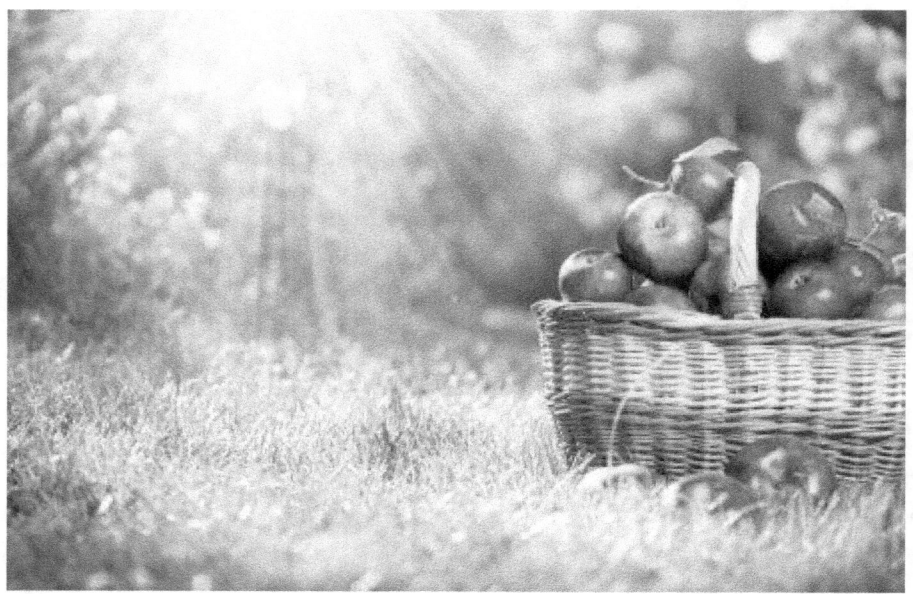

So everybody knows that an apple a day's going to keep the doctor away, but that is really true. This fruit is invaluable in the maintenance of good health and in the prevention and treatment of many ailments. The more sick you are in your youth, the sooner you are going to achieve all age. That is why a healthy diet, right from the very beginning is going to keep you well supplied with plenty of minerals and vitamins.

Apples are also used in alternative medicine to treat anemia, constipation, heart disease, headache, diarrhea, stomach disorders, high blood pressure, rheumatic problems, eye and teeth disorders.

This seems to be quite a long list to us, but our forefathers living millenniums ago suffered from these problems continuously and that is why they made sure that they had plenty of apples included in their daily diets.

The different chemicals which are present in an apple are vitamin B1, phosphorus and potassium. People suffering from lack of memory, lack of concentration, mental depression, mental irritability, and extreme fatigue. I suggested a breakfast of an apple with a glass full of milk with 1 tablespoon full of honey added to it. This is the best pick me up for you physically and mentally.

Apples are considered to be the best fruit to tone up a weak and rundown condition. So if you are prone to ailments, why not boost up your immunity system, as well as your general health by eating lots of apples?

Apples contain more phosphorus and iron than any other vegetable and fruit in older days apples were eaten regularly with the milk to promote good health and the appearance of youthfulness. It also gave you a healthy and excellent skin while relaxing your body and mind.

Cabbages

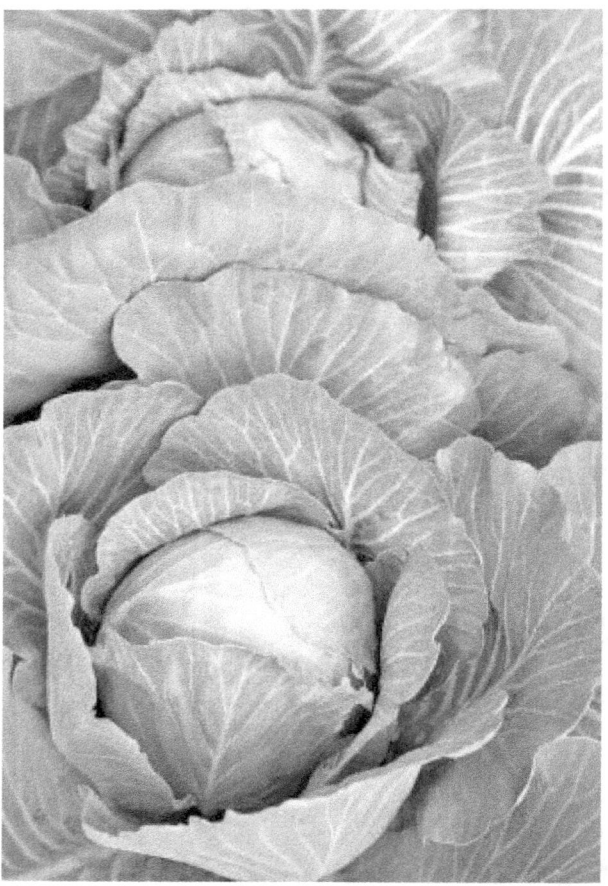

In 18th-century Britain, the aristocrats had stopped eating cabbages, because they considered it the food of the common masses. However, potatoes, cabbages and bacon still continue to be the staple diet of rich and poor in Scotland and Ireland, and no wonder they had better skin, pep and energy, and vitality. This is the difference which one particular vegetable can make in your general health.

This is considered to be the best and most highly rated off leafy vegetables. It cleans up your system and builds muscles. The food value of this widget about includes lots of sulfur and chlorine as well as iodine. This chlorine and sulfur combination cleans up your digestive tract regularly, getting rid of all the accumulated toxins in their. **This is going to happen only when you take cabbage or its juice in its raw state, without adding any salt.**

So the next time you get your hands on a cabbage, pickoff the leaves, wash them to get rid of all the dust and residual pesticides, if any, and begin chomping away like a rabbit. In ancient times, this vegetable was found extremely valuable in constipation, stomach ulcers, skin disorders and obesity.

Cabbages contain several elements and actors which enhance the immunity system of the human body and arrest the premature aging process. That is why the Koreans who knew all about how to arrest signs of aging, made sure that kimchi [1] was a part of one's daily diet. The Germans had sauerkraut. All this is fermented cabbage without any salt added to it.

People suffering from gallbladder problems especially gallstones should increase the intake of cabbage in their diets. Try eating cabbage without salt in its raw form or cooked form.

Skin disorders were cured by applying cabbage juice on pimples, blemishes and other skin problems. This vegetable like cucumber is an excellent cooler of the skin as well as a good moisturizer.

My grandmother kept wrinkles at bay by mixing cabbage juice with honey. Her grandmother had done that, and so on back into the mists of time. So the next time you see your wrinkle appearing on your face, trying mixing up 6 tablespoons full of cabbage juice, with 1 tablespoon full of honey and applying it all over your face. Leave it on until the honey is absorbed. You may want to wash it off, if you think your face is sticky and you are ready to go to sleep. But I normally put this mixture on during the daytime, and leave it on until the skin becomes smooth, silky, well moisturized and youthful looking again.

---

[1] In 1996, Korea got into a dispute with Japan, where manufacturers were selling a product like kimchi, under the name of Kimuchi. This was not fermented cabbage. The original Korean kimchi has Napa cabbage and other ingredients and has to go through a fermentation process.

Honey

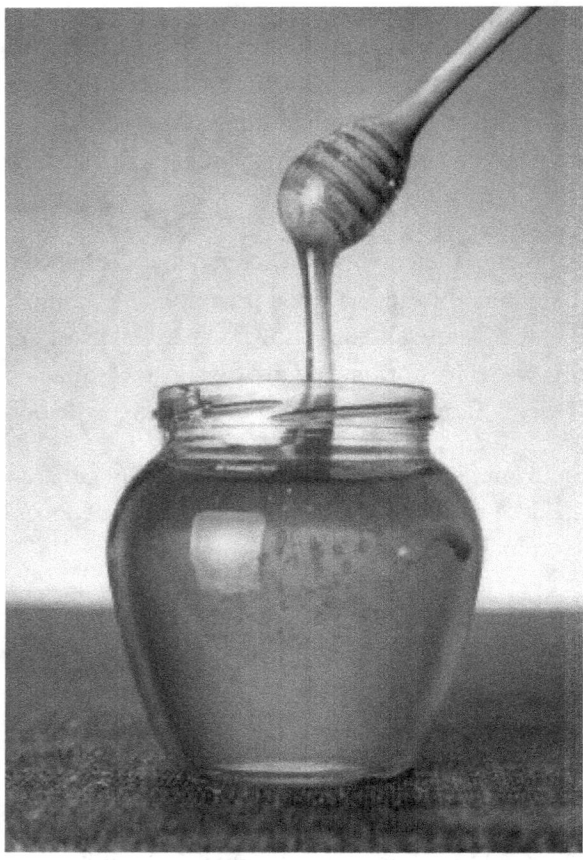

Why was the land full of milk and honey considered to be the ultimate utopia by the ancients? That is because they knew that these two food items would help them, and the future generations survive, and the stock would be healthy forevermore.

Honey is known to possess unique medicinal and nutritional properties. The pollen going up into the making up of honey as the ultimate predigested food has 22 amino acids, 28 minerals, 14 fatty acids, 11 carbohydrates and 11 enzymes.

Honey was used in ancient medicine to cure cough, anemia, pulmonary diseases, insomnia, and stomach disorders.

This is one of the finest sources of energy and heat, and that is why anybody starting to grow old needs to boost up his honey intake. It is also the most easily digested form of carbohydrate, and that is why older people can digest honey without any problem.

Honey enters directly into the bloodstream because of its dextrine content. This is going to provide you with immediate vitality and energy. I remember going through grueling athletic training sessions at university, when we used to come "back to the pavilion" totally wrung out and our trainer handed us pieces of lemon dipped in honey to suck. This immediately refreshed us and also prevented us from getting dehydrated because of sweat loss.

Garlic and onions

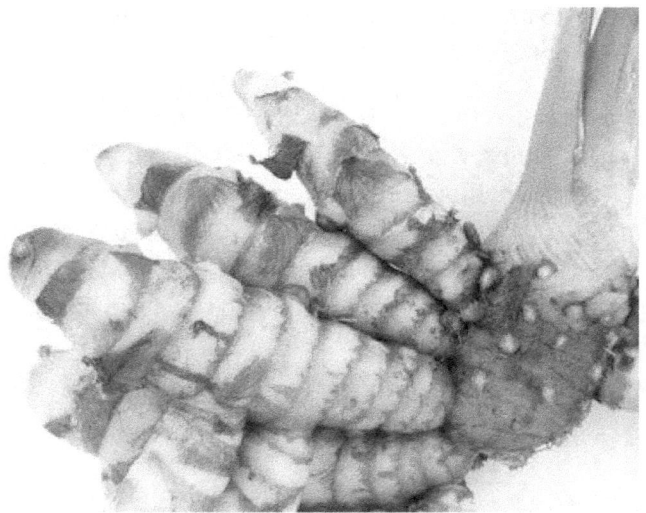

One wonders why garlic began to disappear from British cuisines, just because it had a strong taste around the 17th century, but then the British were never very adventurous about what they ate. Nevertheless, French, Italian, Spanish and other Western cuisine made sure that the garlic and onion content in their daily dishes were added regularly.

This is the reason why onion, which is one of the most versatile and beneficial of natural foods has been used for centuries to cure and prevent ailments. These ailments consisted of influenza, cough, cold, bronchitis, tuberculosis, dropsy, anemia, toothache, earache and so on. This is because onions stimulated the circulation of blood. Onions are a really strong antiseptic, so if you are prone to any infections, increase your onion intake to build up your immunity system.

When we were young, we were given a teaspoonful of fresh onion juice, mixed with a teaspoonful of honey and believe it or not, we never suffered from childhood ailments; except chickenpox, mumps and measles, which we caught during our summer vacations spent in the city and away from the mountains. This says something about living in a polluted atmosphere prone to disease and infections, would not you say?

In many parts of the East as well as in the Middle East, Onions have to be a salad eaten with every meal. This keeps the digestive system working properly. This also adds pep and ginger to your system, as well as makes your food tastier.

If you are suffering from high blood pressure and other problems of the circulatory system, you may want to boil onions and eat them regularly. Do not waste the onion juice obtained after the onion has been boiled. Drink it up without adding any salt or pepper. It is a good intestinal cleanser.

This boiled onion diet is going to reduce the possibility of heart attacks. That is because onions prevent the blood from clotting and thus causing a blockage in the arteries.

Garlic and onions are considered to be as synonymous in the East as bacon and eggs and salt and pepper. Any dish which has onions in it is going to have garlic and ginger added to supplement the taste and nutritional value.

Since ancient times, Garlic was used as a nerve tonic and an excellent therapeutic medicine, thanks to the garlic oil present in it. All over the world, garlic was an important food, for centuries, and the ancient Romans and Egyptians could not do without their daily dose of onions and garlic included in a fish paste.

The original Roman garum sauce eaten as a fermented fish sauce had rudiments of herbs like garlic and onions in it.

In ancient times. Garlic was used to prevent pneumonia, tuberculosis, flatulence, dyspepsia, colds, asthma and bronchitis.

People in the East still believe that the regular use of garlic, even when one is healthy, gives you strength, increases longevity and keeps you fit to work in old age.

In many parts of the East, even today, laborers living below the poverty line dine off bread, onions, garlic and chilies for lunch and survive as their ancestors have been doing for thousands of years. And they are much healthier than their counterparts eating heavy lunches with plenty of fried foods and even junk food.

Sunflower seeds

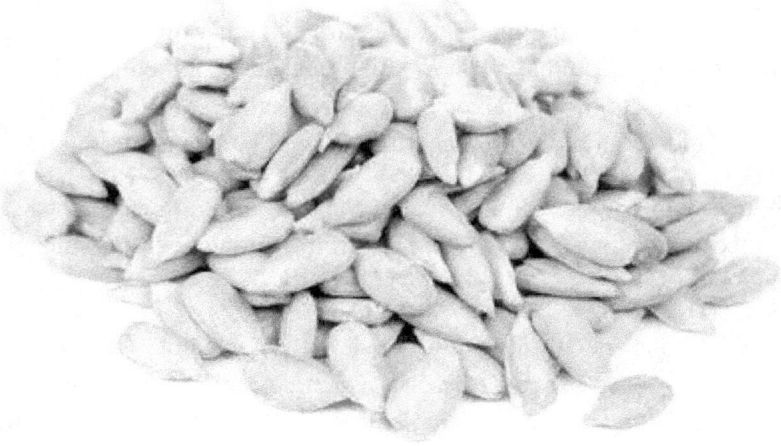

Sunflower seeds are among the most familiar of edible seeds and are available easily all over the world. They have an above-average content of phosphorus, protein, iron, and B complex vitamins. They also have a large percentage of fat which provides one with instant energy, especially if one is feeling lethargic.

You can use these seeds by sprinkling them over salads, cereals, yogurt, soups, and even mixed with vegetables.

They are excellent additions to your diet, especially when you reach your 40s and 50s. That is because they have linoleic acid in them which reduces the cholesterol deposits in your arteries. They also keep your skin, digestive tract, nerve cells and brain cells healthy.

These seeds can help prevent and cure bronchitis, influenza, tonsillitis, cough and other respiratory diseases.

Wheat Sprouts

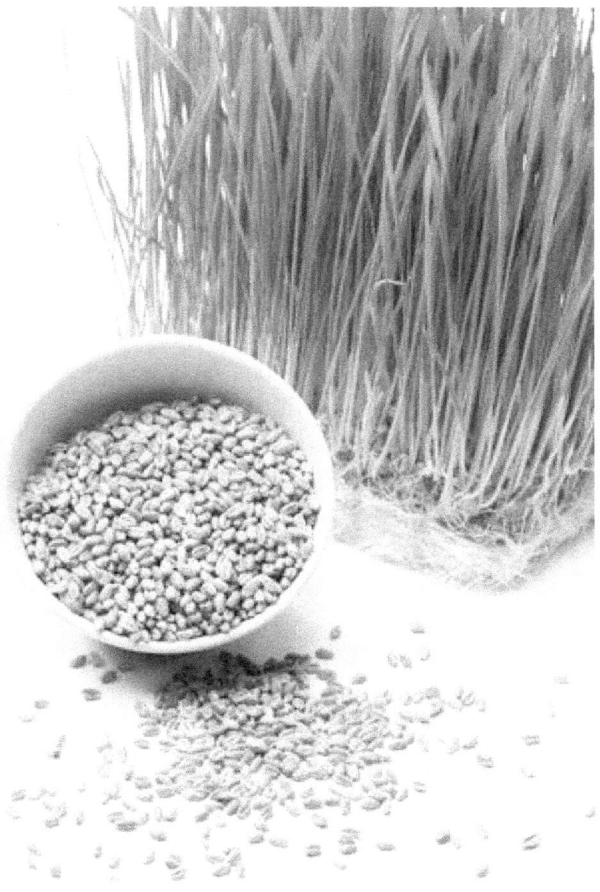

We cannot do without wheat. This precious cereal has been the staple diet of millions who went before us, and it is going to be the most important and widely used serial for making bread, even in the future. This is an excellent source of energy as well as a provider of all those elements necessary to keep a human body working properly.

The gluten and starch content in the wheat is going to provide you with heat and energy. Wheat bran is going to give you mineral salts and phosphates. The outer wheat bran provides you with fiber and roughage to help indigestion and keep your waste and toxin elimination system working properly.

Wheat germs have plenty of protein and vitamin B and E. These help in the building and repairing of muscular tissue. So when you eat whole wheat, which includes ran as well as the wheat, you are going to get natural protection against constipation, heart diseases, diseases of the colon, and thus your life expectancy is going to be prolonged.

Wheatgrass is normally grown by spreading soaked wheat grains in Earth filled earthen pots. They are extremely rich sources of chlorophyll, which can be utilized as a bodybuilder, cleanser and the most beneficial neutralizer of toxins.

Wheatgrass also has a number of minerals. Regular drinking of wheat juice removes toxins from your body. It also maintains good health and prolongs life. This wheat juice is also valuable in the prevention and treatment of skin diseases, digestive system diseases and circulatory disorders. This is because it strengthens up your metabolism and autoimmune system, and furnishes your body with required nourishment and extra energy.

Yogurt

In ancient times pure milk products like butter, butter milk and yogurt were considered to be very necessary additions in one's daily diet in order to keep healthy and youthful looking. Women used to bathe in buttermilk to prevent wrinkles. They also washed their hair in yogurt to prevent premature grayness. Of course, that left one smelling rancid, but in different times, different odors were considered normal, because everyone around one smelled just like you!

Yogurt or as it is commonly called curd or curds is a lactic fermentation of milk. It is a highly versatile and health promoting food. It is also very valuable as a therapeutic food item given to patients as well as to healthy people. In order to promote good health, you need to have yogurt at least twice a day with meals.

I remember having a meal with a traditional family and sweet yogurt was placed on each platter. And the family members demanded more helpings of this yogurt. The cook was glad to provide this particular healthy food to all of them because according to her, a constant and regular use of yogurt kept the intestinal tract, happy and healthy. She did not have to bother about constipation or tummy problems in such cases.

The yogurt which you buy in the market has preservatives. That's why you may want to make your own yogurt. Yogurt makers are easily available in the market, but I would suggest an earthenware pot, which can be used for cooking. Try boiling milk in this pot , and you never boil it again in any other metal utensil ever.

You can then make yogurt in this clay pot.

Making yogurt the traditional way is not very hard, but you need a yogurt starter. If you have not made yogurt before, take a spoonful of yogurt from one of the store bought simple yogurt products without any additions. Once you have made yogurt with this starter, you can continue making yogurt umpteen times, with just one spoonful of the yogurt starter left over from your previous yogurt session.

How to Make Traditional Yogurt

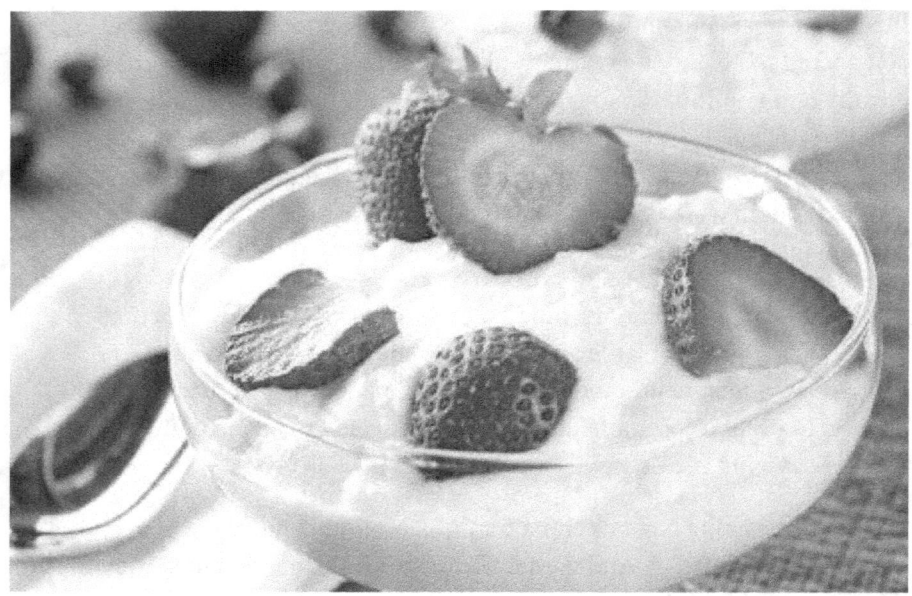

You make yogurt in the East in this traditional way. Normally, milk is boiled in many parts of the East, even though you may get it pasteurized. Because traditionally, people in the East do not trust the pasteurizing process and would rather boil it again before use, than drink it straight from the milk bottle or from the packet.

So boil 1 L of milk. Allow to cool until it is lukewarm. You are going to see a thin layer of cream floating on top. You can keep it to add some taste you are making yogurt.

You need 3 tablespoons full of yogurt culture. What is yogurt culture? It is just the remainder of the yogurt, which was left behind after you finished the yogurt you made yesterday. Remember to keep at least 2 to 3 tablespoons full and do not empty out that yogurt bowl.

Dip your finger in the milk. If it is tolerably warm, in warm weather, this is the time you put in the yogurt. Whip it briskly with a spoon, cover with a lid, and placed by one side of the stove in your warm kitchen. This is normally made overnight, so that you have perfect yogurt to eat for breakfast the next morning. The next morning, it has set, so put it in the fridge.

If you really want a traditional taste, boil this milk in a red earthenware pot, allow it to cool to lukewarm, add the culture, and leave the yogurt to set. This is considered to be one of the most delicious ways in which to eat milk products and meat products in India, and also in other countries in the East – cooking in earthenware pots. This yogurt is going to have the taste of mother Earth, in a sweetened form.

I still cannot understand how that yogurt got sweet. I never added any sugar to it. It is also going to have a distinctly delicious wet earthenware aroma.

Also, I found a friend setting yogurt in cold weather, – freezing Missouri weather – by warming up her oven at 125°C for five minutes. Then she put in the yogurt container in the oven and left it overnight. Good idea!

This yogurt is excellent for eating on its own, as a dip, or as an accompaniment. You can also use it as a marinade for meat. Churn it to make butter and buttermilk.

Traditional Buttermilk

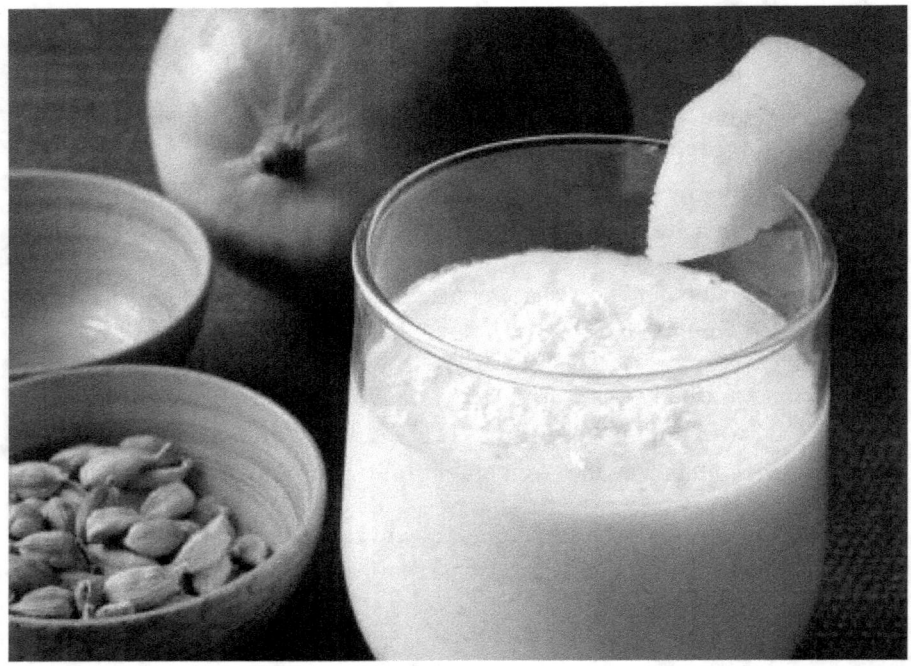

This buttermilk has mango pulp added.

The buttermilk that you buy in the store is not purely traditional, because it has been pasteurized, and it has been homogenized. People in the West normally considered that to be "real" buttermilk, but in the East, buttermilk is a made up of churning pure butter. That butter is made by churning cream with water. You can also get this butter by churning yogurt with water.

What Are the Health Benefits of Buttermilk?

Apart from its being a really refreshing drink, it is a really delicious digestive. It is normally drunk on its own, or with the little bit of rock salt and pepper added to it with a couple of mint leaves just for show. Or you may want to add honey. Many traditional medicines are given to the patients, with buttermilk instead of water. This buttermilk is salty and is called *matha*.

In ancient Ayurveda treatments, milk products, including buttermilk, butter and yogurt were used extensively, to give plenty of strength to patients as well as to encourage a healthy nutritional supplement to normal, healthy folk. They also were known to provide longevity.

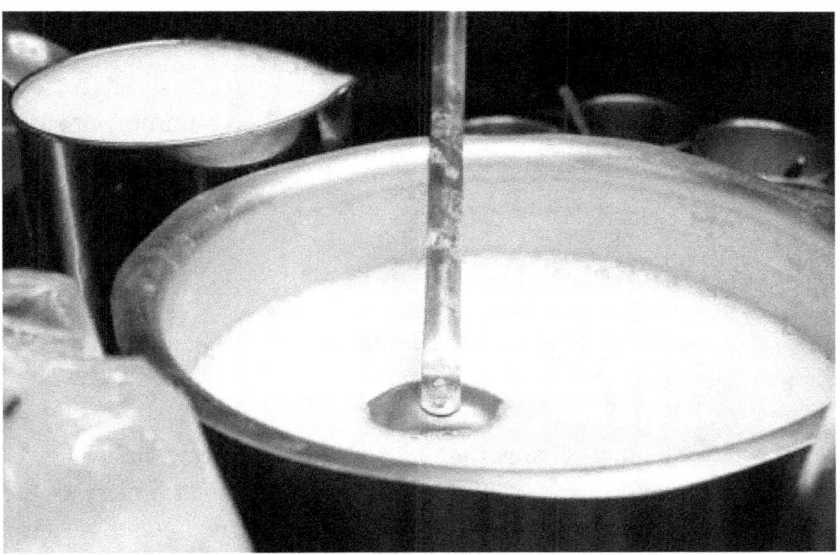

How Do You Make Traditional Buttermilk?

2 cups rich creamy yogurt.
2 Equal amount of crushed ice or iced water.
Two table spoons honey – if you want it sweet.
Pepper and salt to taste
Half a teaspoonful of roasted roughly ground cumin seeds – if you want it salty

Since ancient times in the East, when there were no mixers and blenders around, all these items were placed in a huge churn and churned by hand until the mixture was frothy. The side product was of course fresh butter, which would then be scooped off and placed in clay containers.

This buttermilk was then topped off with a slice of cream or yogurt and served as an excellent digestive, with lunch in summer, or just drunk whenever you feel thirsty, to prevent you from getting dehydrated in the hot summer sun.

Digestive Buttermilk

This is normally drunk with every meal. It helps in the digestion. It also keeps you really healthy.

For this you need 2 cups of water, half a cup of plain yogurt, half a teaspoonful of cumin seeds, or powdered cumin seeds, 1 inch piece of fresh ginger, one tablespoonful of cilantro/mint leaves, chopped up into pieces, and pinch of salt.

Put all the ingredients together except the cilantro into a blender and blend until the buttermilk is foamy. Garnish with cilantro and put in the jug, so that your whole family can pour it out, when they have finished their lunch or dinner. If you want sweet buttermilk, you can add 2 tablespoons of honey. Once I put in half a teaspoonful of ground cardamom and half a teaspoonful of fresh grated ginger in this buttermilk and found it really refreshing and tasty. That was spicy buttermilk!

Salty Buttermilk

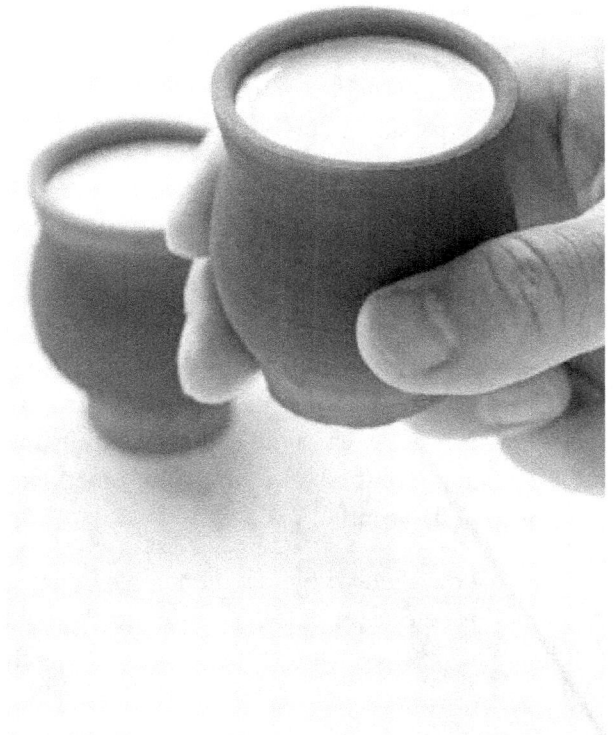

Any milk products which you buy in India, including buttermilk or yogurt is always placed in these clay cups. They enhance the taste and are eco-friendly, because one does not bother about plastic packaging.

This is one item, which is definitely not ignored by people living in the North, South and Western parts of the Indian subcontinent. It is named with local names, but it is the same – spiced and salty buttermilk. It is drunk as often as possible with lunch as their digestive accompaniment, instead of water. In such cases, it is sprinkled with a mixture of powdered roasted cumin seeds and roasted curry leaves, rock salt, pepper, cayenne pepper, and just this little pinch of asafoetida.

One takes a healthy swallow, and is grateful for the refreshing spicy feeling. This is an acquired taste, because it is going to be slightly sour in taste. That is because of the fermented bacteria, which are sold to you in supermarkets under the name of probiotic drinks.

All those are nothing but homemade buttermilk made up of Stale yogurt, packaged expensively and marketed winningly with scientific terms like probiotic bacteria, amazingly good for your health and all those impressive statements made by the superstar endorsing them on TV.

This is what happened when it came to India for the first time. People went crazy, because it was something new, and had been "discovered" by a company who hired one of India's most popular superstars to endorse it.Yakult, it is good for your gut.

 So people bought, they drank and said, "hey, what a sell! [No pun intended.] We are buying our own buttermilk and yogurt under the name of probiotic bacteria. And it is not even salted and spiced. Whattabore!"And went home, and asked their moms or wives to churn something really traditional in the shape of buttermilk.

Those products went off the shelf within the month. No other company has turned up with probiotic bacteria products, because they know that they are not going to sell in the land, where butter, buttermilk and yogurt is still churned by hand.

Spicy Salt

Naturally, you are not going to drink it without a mixture of spices. The spices are going to include **2 teaspoons full of powdered and roasted cumin seeds, one teaspoonful of black salt, 1 teaspoon of rocksalt, half a teaspoonful of pepper, and a handful of powdered dried mint leaves.** Grind all of them together and put them into your favorite pepper shaker.

Whenever you need to spice up your buttermilk, just sprinkle, stir, and drink. The mint and cumin seeds are going to help in your digestion, especially in the summer.

This spicy salt can also be used as a sprinkle on salads and also on yogurt or sandwich mixes and yogurt-based dips.

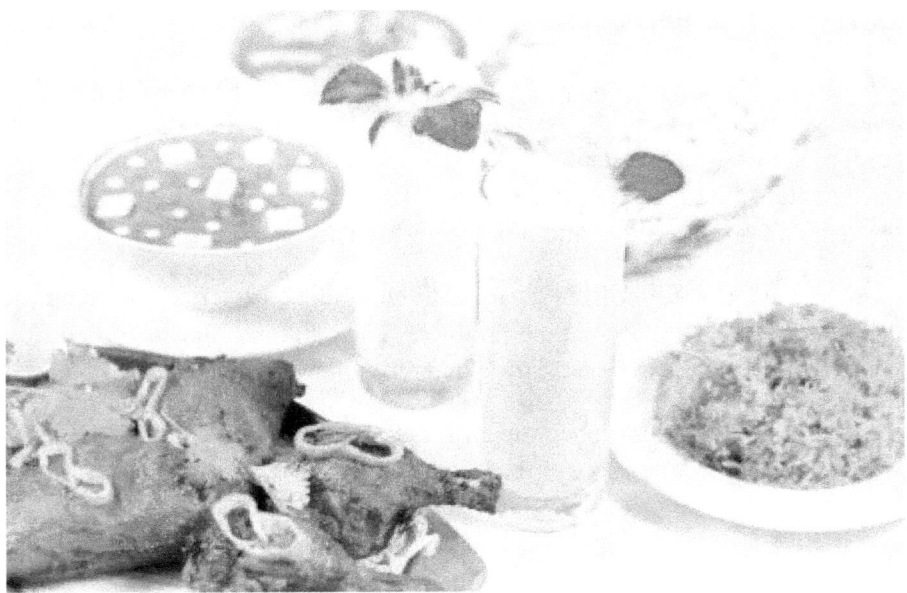

So the next time you are eating chicken tandoori, ask the restaurateur-where is my lassi? You are going to be given a choice of sweet, salty, flavored [with fruit pulp] or plain.

Making Butter Out Of Cream

The top cream layer, on boiled milk is collected, and allowed to keep for a couple of days, so that the probiotic bacteria can flourish in them. So the day, when you want to make fresh butter, you take all this cream, and put it in the blender with some water. The water is going to separate, and you are going to have lumps of unsalted butter.

Can you make butter from fresh cream? Yes you can, but you are going to note the different quality of the butter made from "stale" cream, as compared to fresh cream butter. That is because fresh cream does not have many lactic acid bacteria in it, yet. But as it is, that cream is going to ferment and produce more and more lactic bacteria.

Also, if you make butter from cream with more lactic bacteria, it is going to increase the shelf life of the final product. That is because the bacteria do not allow any other bacteria to grow in their vicinity.

Buttermilk in the Indian subcontinent is the liquid, which is left over after the cream and the yogurt are churned with water.

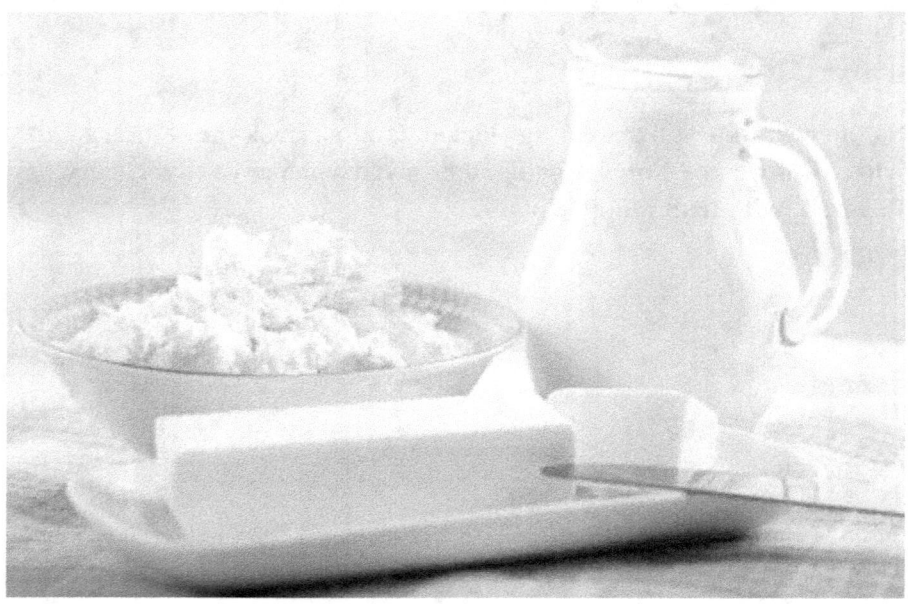

The crumbly white food item is pure homemade white butter, while the solid chunky square is cottage cheese.

Traditional Clarified Butter – Desi Ghee

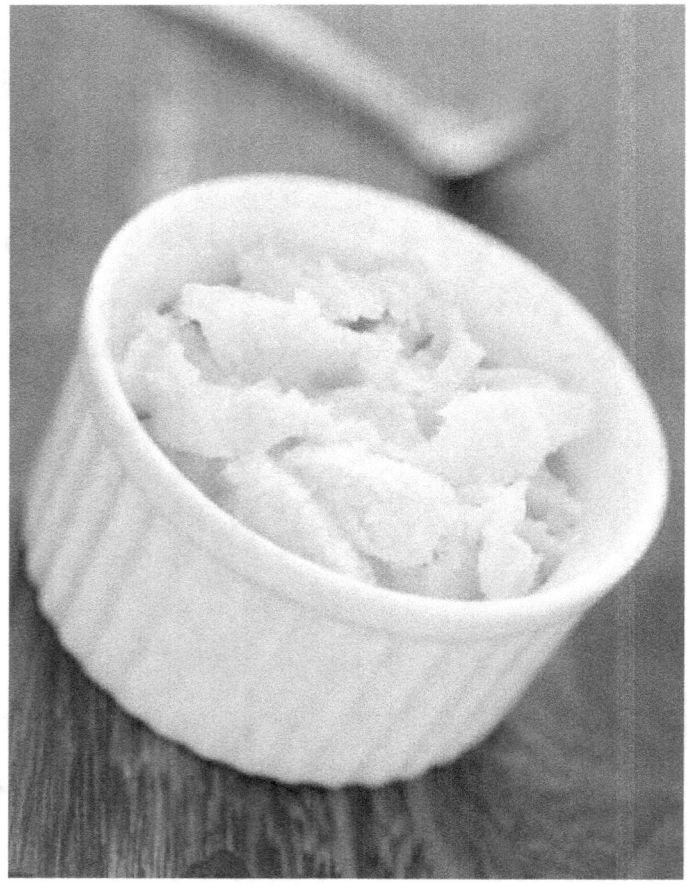

Desi ghee is clarified butter, which is extremely concentrated and a very powerful healing agent. It is normally used in the making up of herbal medicines, because it is made of pure creamy milk butter. It is also used in making beauty creams, potions, lotions and other skin ointments.

It has a powerful aroma, and that is why only just a spoonful is added to fry meats. It is going to float on the surface of the meat dish, after it has been cooked, so you need to stir the gravy before serving. Also, the food is not going to taste greasy, even though it looks like it has been swimming in fat.

Desi ghee is the concentrated form of pure butter, which is heated to reduce the butter of all the impurities as well as moisture. This concentrated butter is normally used in Eastern cuisine, for searing meat, sautéing and frying food, because they offer its higher burning point. You make this at home by taking 2 pounds of best unsalted butter and melting it in a heavy bottomed pan. Allow the butter to liquefy on low heat for about 40 minutes. Maintain this simmering point, until all of the moisture in the butter has evaporated. The impurities are going to sink to the bottom of the pan. Remember to keep stirring the butter, so that it does not burn.

Pour off the clear butter and strain it through several thicknesses of muslin cloth. This butter is going to last for about a year, if it is placed in a cool and dry place. This butter is exorbitantly expensive. So in the East, people with easy access to plenty fresh milk make it right in their kitchens for crisp delicious frying results, and adding that taste of pure butter to all their dishes.

A spoonful of this rich concentrated clarified butter eaten every day with your meals would keep you healthy and energetic. Ancient medicine always is made up of herbs in clarified butter. As this butter is the most concentrated form of milk, it is eaten in small quantities, just for its flavor, nutritive value and beneficial properties.

Conclusion

This book gives you some introductory knowledge to naturopathy, and how it helps in longevity. It is a matter what your age is; you may want to come back to nature right now. Stop using chemical-based drugs and start upon a natural diet full of green fruit and vegetables. There are some food items, which hasten the aging process. These include refined white bread, white sugar and polished rice. Similarly, excessive consumption of tea and coffee is injurious to health and leads to weakening of your system.

You need 10 – 15 g of salt daily depending on the climate and occupation of the diner. However, a number of us enjoy lots of salt in our food. Even though salt is a major factor needed to maintain the acid and basic equilibrium of the body, and also for the working of various muscles and nerves, excess of salt can undermine your general health. This excess salt is going to put an extra burden on your kidneys and may cause high blood pressure.

High salt content foods include salted nuts, biscuits, meat, fish, chicken, eggs, cheese, dried fruits, spinach, carrot and horseradish. Low-sodium foods include sugar, cereals, fresh fruit, and honey, peas, onions, potatoes, cabbage, cauliflower, tomatoes and pumpkins.

Doctors who tell you to stop eating salt totally and immediately made do you more harm in the long run because it is necessary to keep your body functioning properly. So you need to add a very small quantity of salt, sprinkled on the dish after cooking just for taste. This is just going to be enough to satisfy your taste buds without harming your body. An excessive intake of salt is capable of leading to stomach problems, hardening of arteries, stomach ulcers, and heart diseases.

Now that you have got some informative and interesting information about different ways and means in which people stayed healthy and youthful looking in ancient times, remember that it is all due to nature and natural foods.

So come back to nature. Live Long and Prosper!

Clay Pot Cookery[2]

It is a well-known fact that the ancients in the East used clay utensils in which to cook their food. This food lasted even longer, than the food, which was cooked in other metal utensils. 4000 years ago clay pots were used to cook everything, all over the world. Even today wise-men well-versed in ancient lore recommends clay pot cookery because the micronutrients present in the clay are exactly what your body needs.

Some people are under the impression that it is going to take longer to cook a meal in a clay pot, when compared to that same dish cooked in a metal pressure cooker or Wok or pan. That is not true. The capacity of the vessel is the same, the source of heat is the same. It is only the material going up into the making of the cooking pot, which is different.

If you are using a clay pot for the first time, or even earthenware, wash it out properly, and boil some water in it. This is going to remove the clay smell. After that dry the pots in the sun.

When dry, you need to temper your cooking pot by pouring some oil into it. Then heat it well. This procedure "seals" the cooking pot, and prevents it from cracking – unless of course you allow it to slip from your hands and smash onto the kitchen floor.

So if you find a place where you can get a clay pot and you want to start cooking in it, come back to nature and try this now. Steaming, frying, roasting, boiling, and slow cooking can be done in this clay pot. The natural

---

[2] http://www.amazon.com/Indian-Clay-Biriyani-Pot-Medium/dp/B00OYX9HOY.

This is what it looks like. Naturally, my pots are unglazed, because I bought them from the friendly neighborhood roadside Potter. It is called a Handi. They are very common in the east, but in the West, you have to rely on amazon or on a company selling you a glazed product.

clay, which makes up the pot helps keep you healthy because of the calcium, phosphorus and magnesium content present in the clay.[3]

Many people may consider eating out of a clay pot to be barbaric, because hey, according to them, it is unhygienic. One does not know about the clay which has been used in the making of this pot. Funnily enough, we have our own mindsets, and would limit our diets as well as naturopathic cures, because the ingredients and cooking methods according to us are strange and weird.

The earthenware pots that you get on eBay are going to be around $105. Do not buy them because they are glazed. And expensive.

---

[3] https://www.youtube.com/watch?v=pW0KcySGN_k shows you a slide show on how a woman uses this pots on her gas burner. Keep the Flame low or medium.

Author Bio

Dueep Jyot Singh is a Management and IT Professional who managed to gather Postgraduate qualifications in Management and English and Degrees in Science, French and Education while pursuing different enjoyable career options like being an hospital administrator, IT,SEO and HRD Database Manager/ trainer, movie , radio and TV scriptwriter, theatre artiste and public speaker, lecturer in French, Marketing and Advertising, ex-Editor of Hearts On Fire (now known as Solstice) Books Missouri USA, advice columnist and cartoonist, publisher and Aviation School trainer, ex-moderator on Medico.in, banker, student councilor ,travelogue writer … among other things!

One fine morning, she decided that she had enough of killing herself by Degrees and went back to her first love -- writing. It's more enjoyable! She already has 48 published academic and 14 fiction- in- different- genre books under her belt.

When she is not designing websites or making Graphic design illustrations for clients , she is browsing through old bookshops hunting for treasures, of which she has an enviable collection – including R.L. Stevenson, O.Henry, Dornford Yates, Maurice Walsh, De Maupassant, Victor Hugo, Sapper, C.N. Williamson, "Bartimeus" and the crown of her collection- Dickens "The Old Curiosity Shop," and so on… Just call her "Renaissance Woman") - collecting herbal remedies, acting like Universal Helping Hand/Agony Aunt, or escaping to her dear mountains for a bit of exploring, collecting herbs and plants and trekking.

Check out some of the other JD-Biz Publishing books

Gardening Series on Amazon

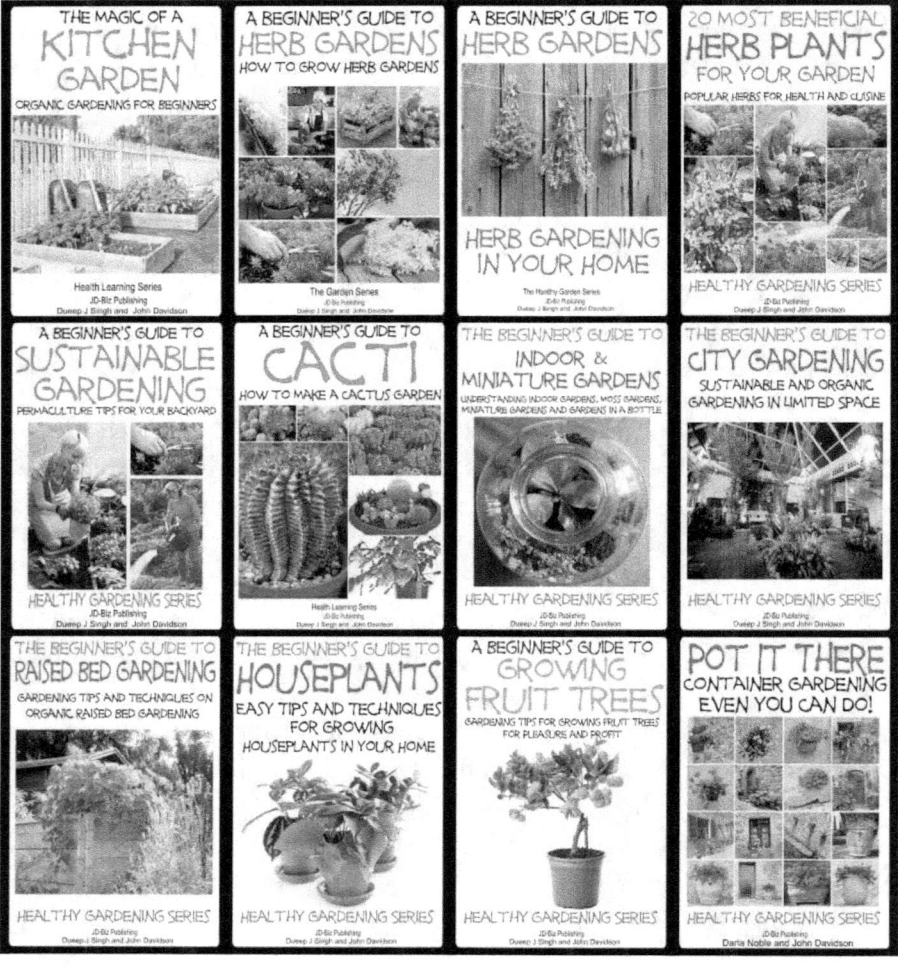

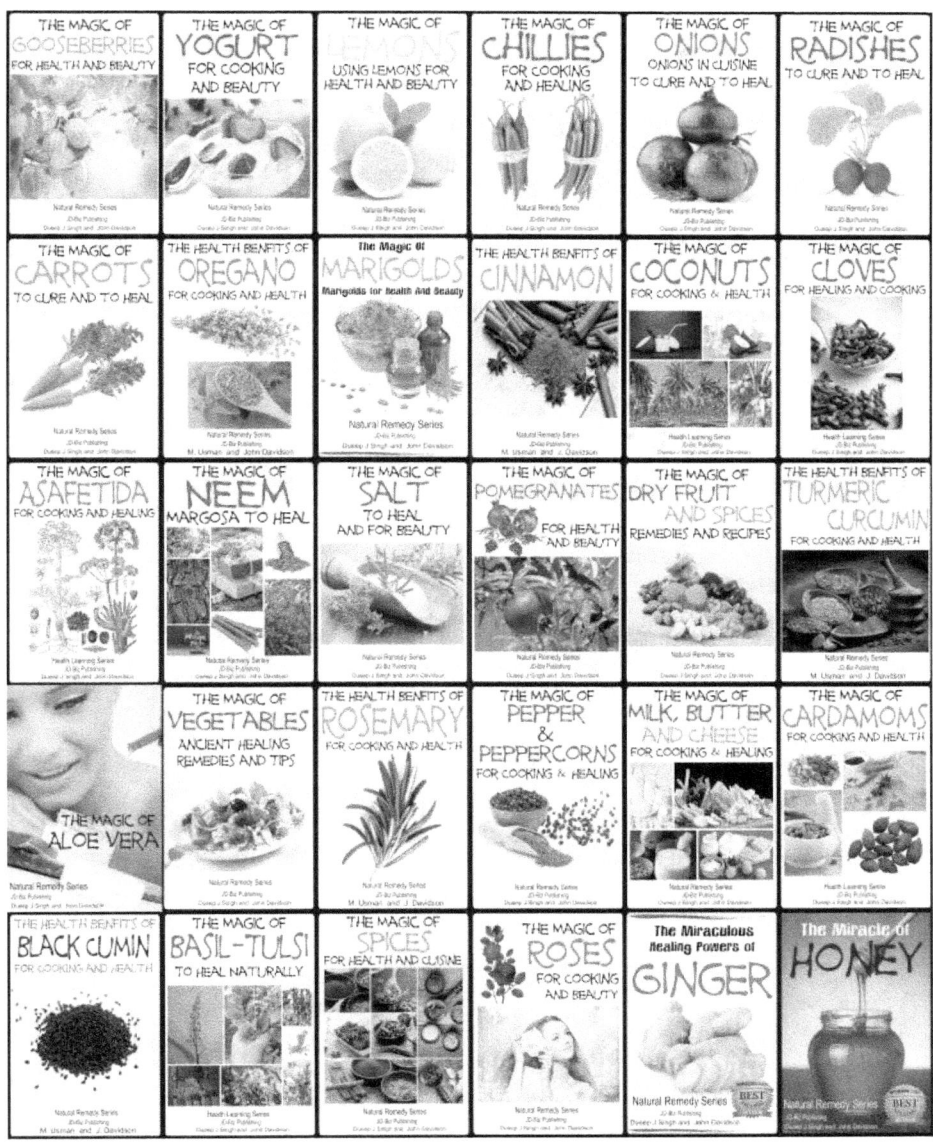

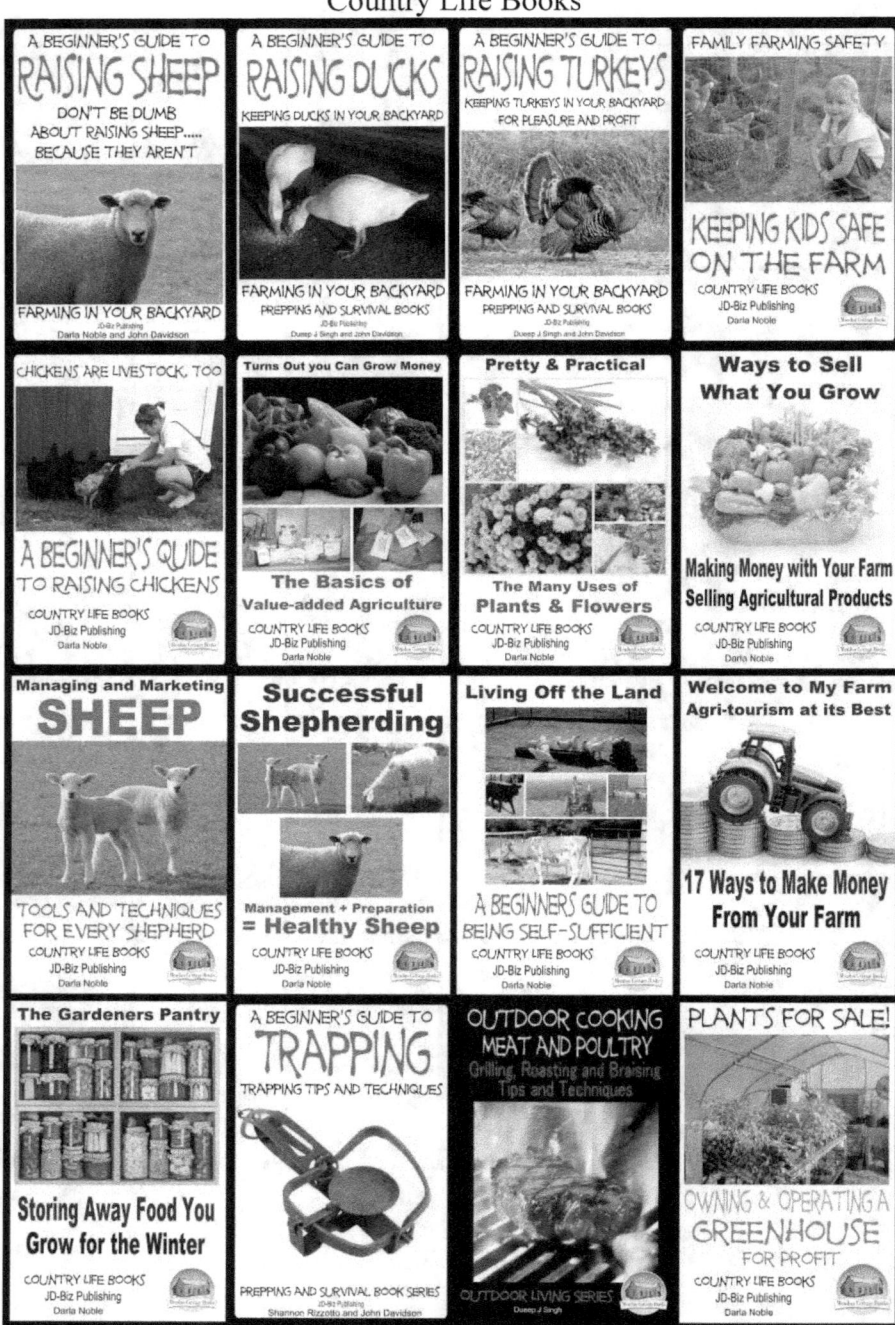

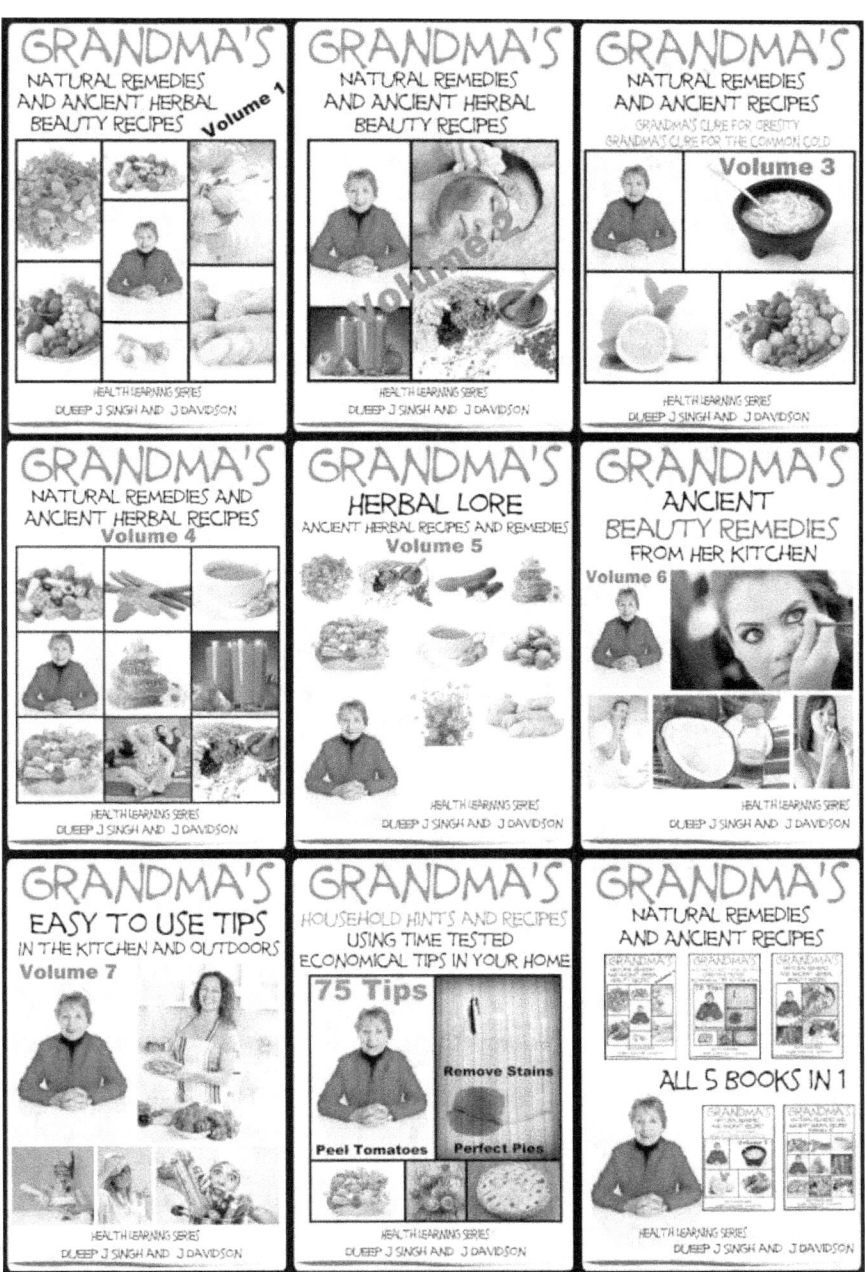

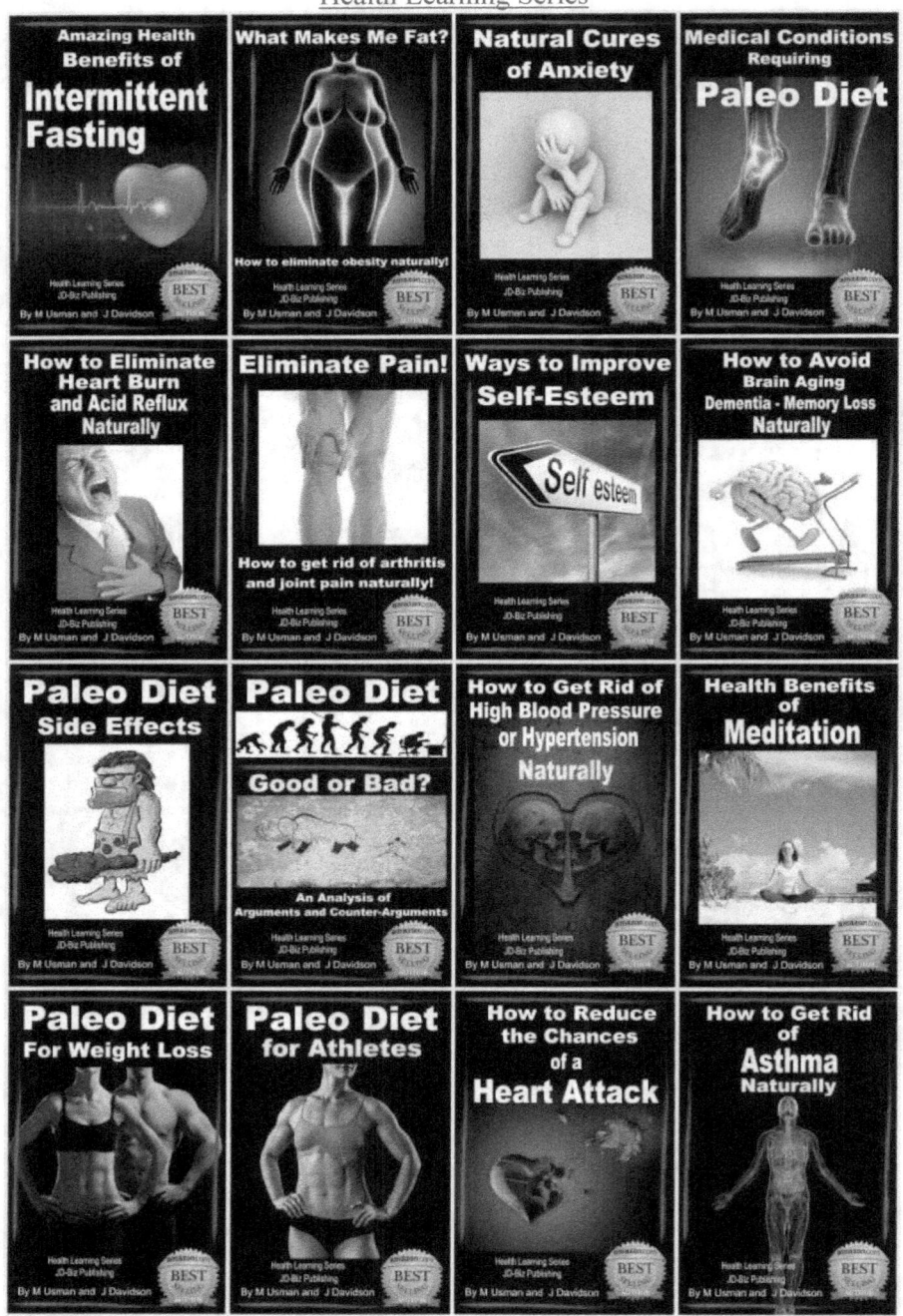

Amazing Animal Book Series

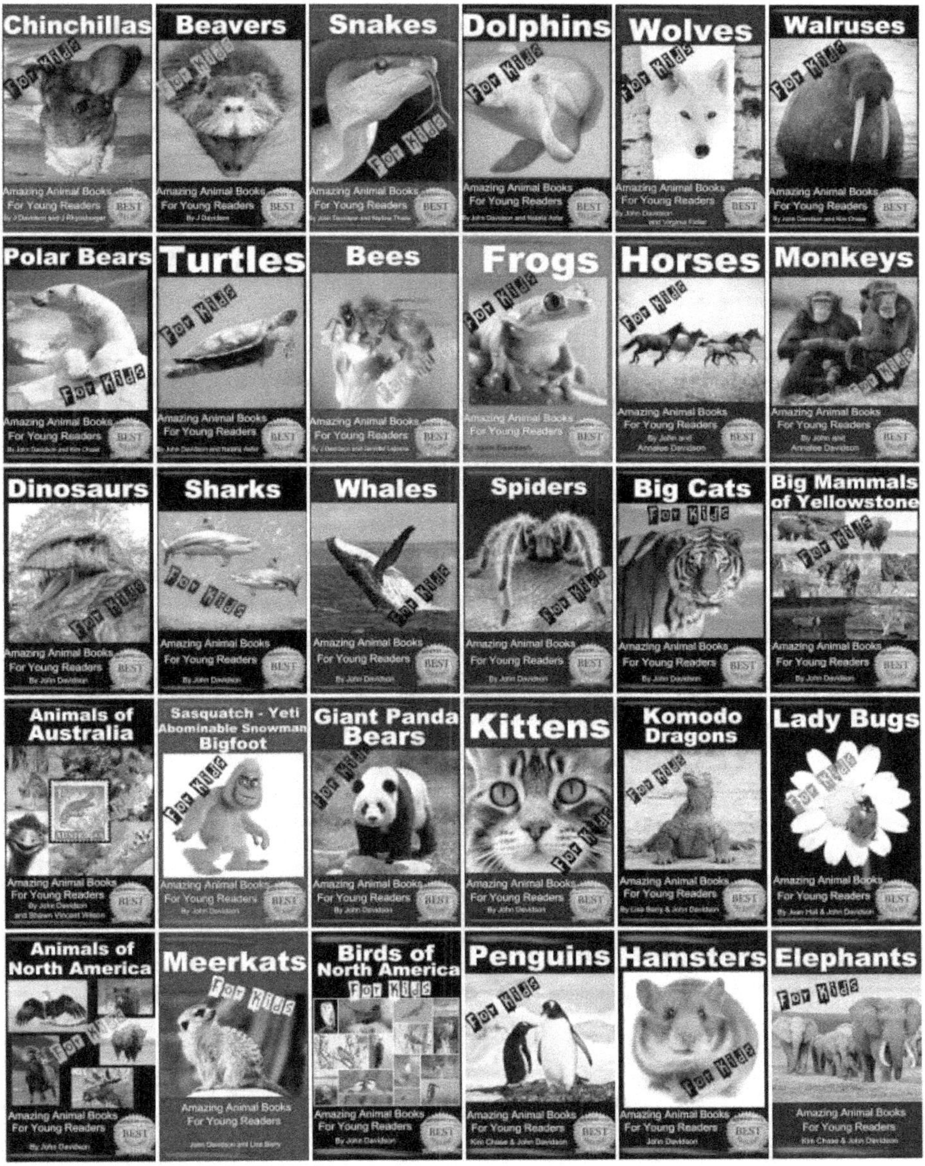

Learn To Draw Series

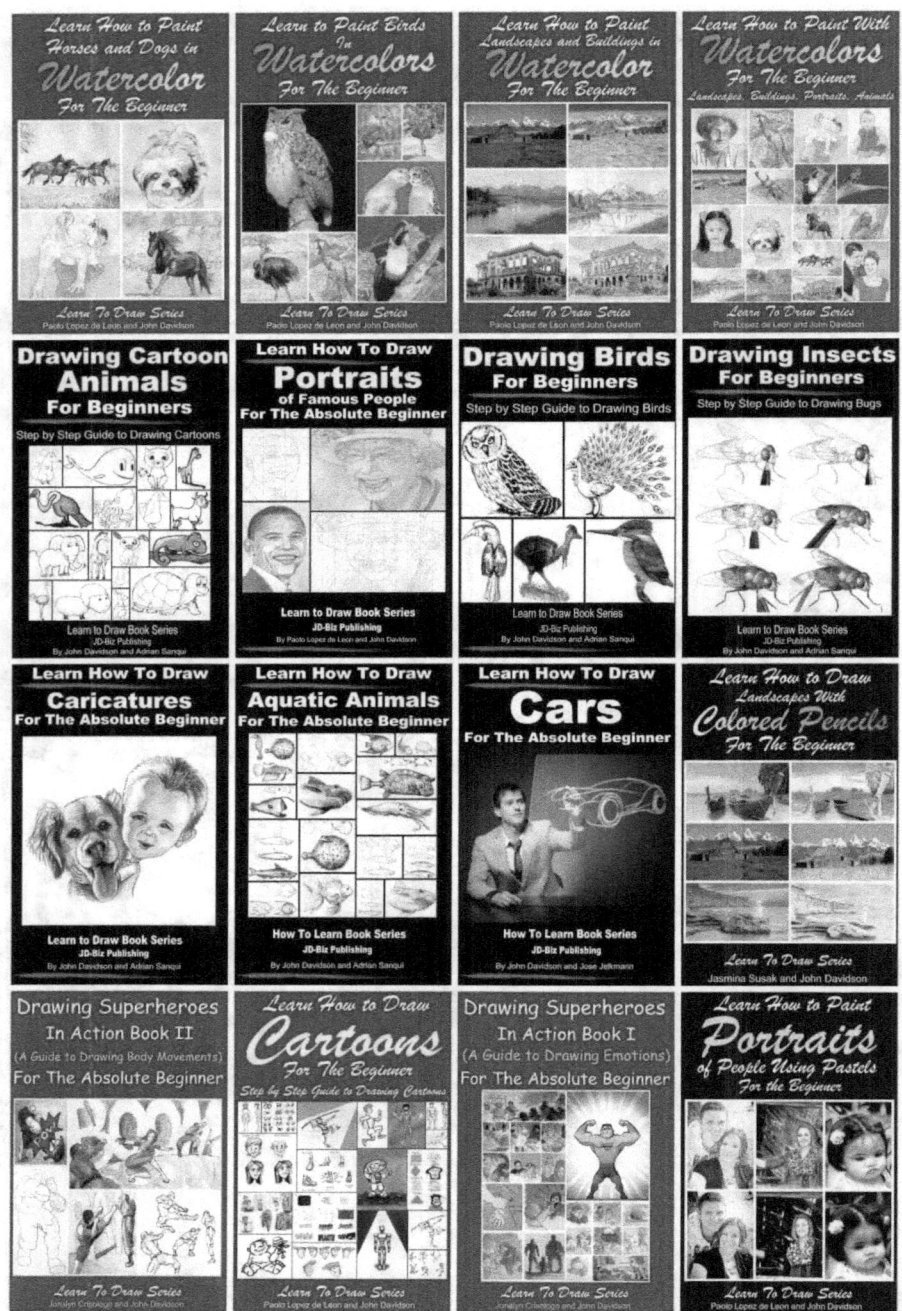

How to Build and Plan Books

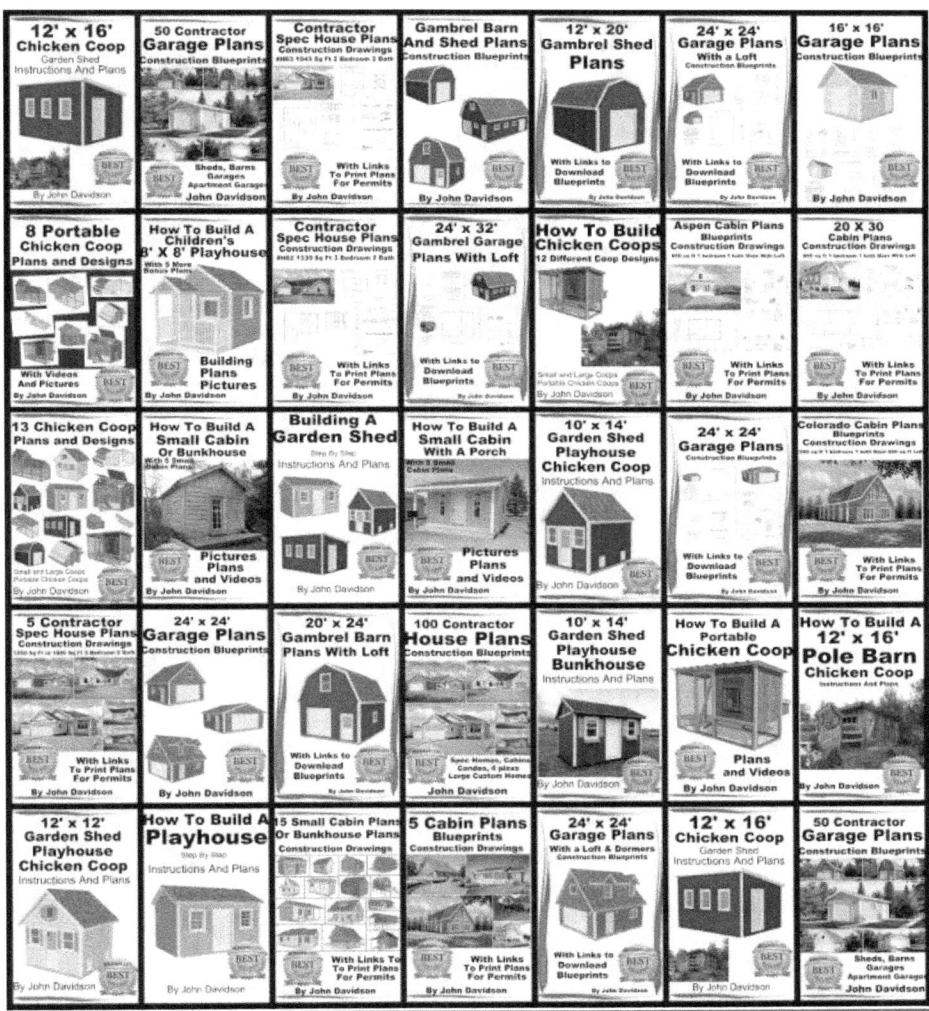

Entrepreneur Book Series

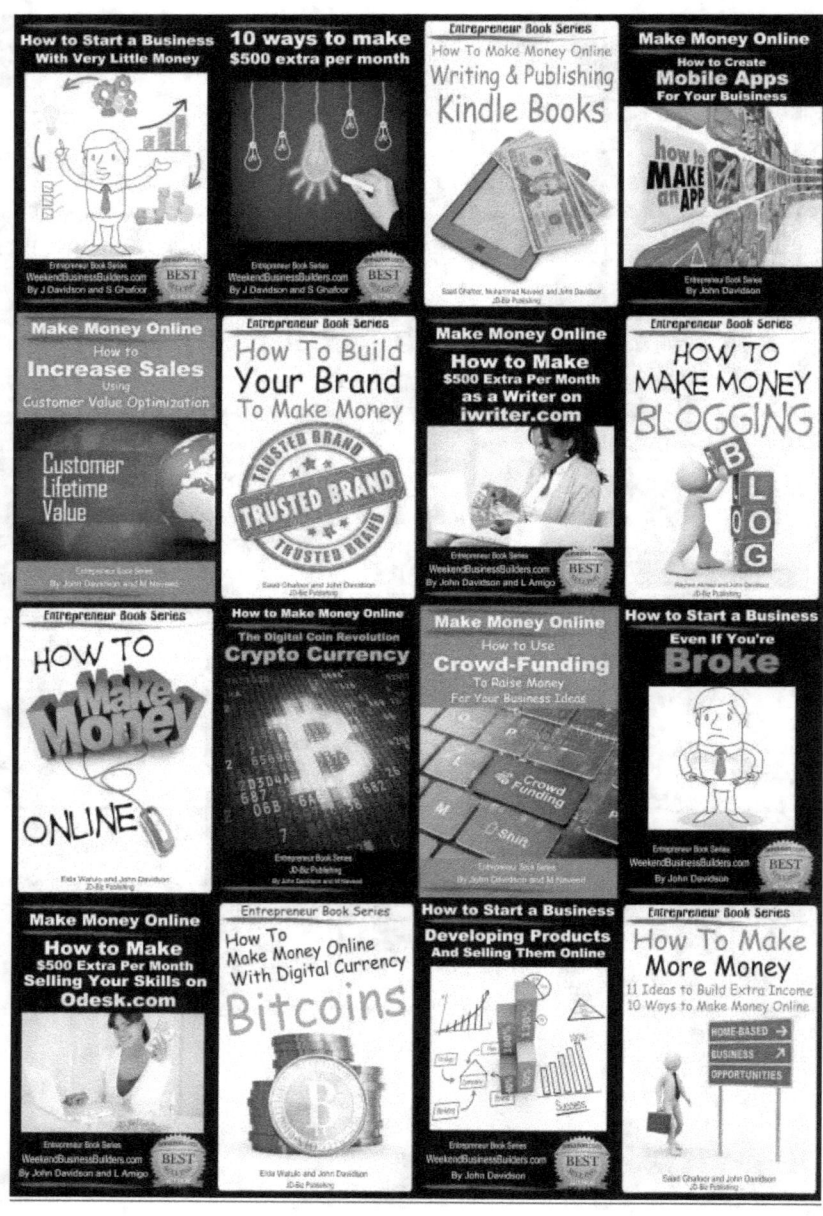

Our books are available at

1. Amazon.com

2. Barnes and Noble

3. Itunes

4. Kobo

5. Smashwords

6. Google Play Books

Publisher

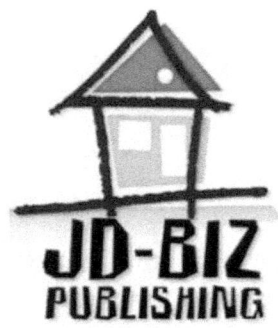

JD-Biz Corp

P O Box 374

Mendon, Utah 84325

http://www.jd-biz.com/

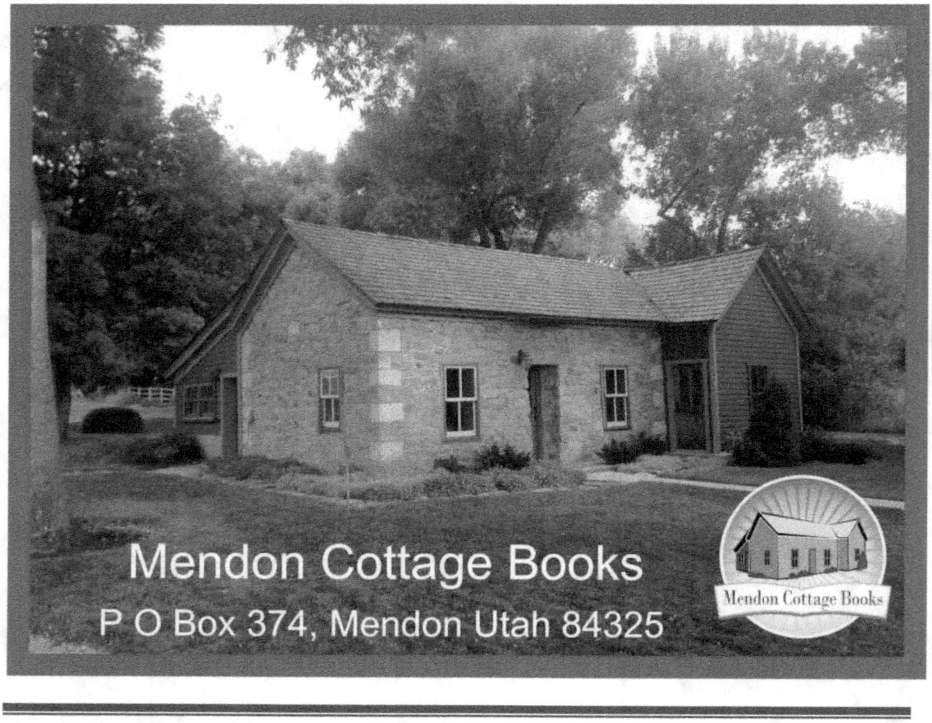

Mendon Cottage Books

P O Box 374, Mendon Utah 84325

www.ingramcontent.com/pod-product-compliance
Lightning Source LLC
Chambersburg PA
CBHW071122280526
45787CB00003B/1136